TABLE OF CONTENTS**

- Arm Circles

- Ankle Rolls

4. **Strength Exercises**

1. **Chair Squats**

   - Instructions

   - Modifications

2. **Wall Push-Ups**

   - Instructions

   - Modifications

3. **Toe Stands**

   - Instructions

   - Modifications

5. **Balance Exercises**

1. **Heel-to-Toe Walk**

- Instructions

- Safety Tips

2. **Standing Leg Lifts**

- Instructions

- Safety Tips

6. **Flexibility Exercises**

1. **Seated Side Stretch**

- Instructions

2. **Upper Body Stretch**

- Instructions

7. **Cool Down Exercises**

- Gentle Walking in Place

- Seated Forward Bend

- Neck Stretch

8. **Maintaining Your Routine**

- Tracking Your Progress

- Setting Realistic Goals

*Bonus advise and more exercises that you can work towards For those seniors above average

9. **FAQs**

10. **Acknowledgments**

11. **About the Author**

Foreword

Welcome to "Easy and Safe Home Exercises for Seniors," a guide specifically designed to help seniors maintain their physical strength and mobility from the comfort of their own home. This book is filled with easy-to-follow exercises that have been tailored for seniors looking to improve their physical health without the need for specialized gym equipment. Before starting any exercise regimen, it's important to consult with a healthcare provider to ensure these activities are suitable for your individual health status.

Safety First

Before we dive into the exercises, it's paramount to prioritize safety to prevent injury. Ensure you have a clear space free from obstacles, wear comfortable clothing and supportive shoes, and always keep water nearby to stay hydrated. Remember, if at any point an exercise feels painful or uncomfortable, stop immediately and consult with a healthcare professional.

Lets Began With A Few Warm-Up Exercises: Shoulder

1. Stand or sit with your back straight and shoulders relaxed.

2. Roll your shoulders slowly in a forward circular motion for 10-15 seconds.

3. Reverse the direction and roll your shoulders backward for another 10-15 seconds.

4. This exercise helps to loosen the shoulders and neck, preparing your body for more strenuous activity.

2nd Warm Up Balance Exercises: Heel-to-Toe Walk

1. Find a flat and unobstructed path in your home.

2. Position the heel of one foot in front of the toes of the opposite foot each time you take a step. Imagine you are walking on a tightrope.

3. Extend your arms to help maintain balance and focus on a steady point in front of you to aid concentration and stability.

4. Walk 10 steps forward, then carefully turn around and walk back.

This book aims to empower seniors to maintain and improve their physical health safely at home. Each exercise comes with step-by-step instructions and modifications to accommodate varying fitness levels. Remember, consistency is key, so try to incorporate these exercises into your daily routine for the best results. Stay active, stay safe, and most importantly, have fun!

Chapter One : Ending Warm-Up Exercises

PART 1. STRETCHING

Exercise 1 : Head Tilts

1. **Start Position**: Sit or stand up straight with your shoulders relaxed, and your hands resting comfortably at your sides.

2. **Movement**: Gently tilt your head towards your right shoulder, aiming to bring your ear closer to the shoulder without raising the shoulder.

3. **Hold**: Keep this position for 10-15 seconds, feeling a stretch on the opposite side of your neck.

4. **Return**: Slowly bring your head back to the center.

5. **Repeat**: Perform the same movement on the left side. Complete 3-5 times for each side.

Exercise 2 : Shoulder Rolls

1. **Start Position**: Stand or sit with your back straight and arms by your sides.

2. **Movement**: Lift your shoulders up towards your ears in a shrugging motion.

3. **Roll**: Roll your shoulders back, bringing your shoulder blades together, and then down.

4. **Reverse**: After completing a few backward rolls, switch to forward rolls.

5. **Repeat**: Do 10-15 rolls in each direction.

Exercise 3 : Arm Circles

1. **Start Position**: Stand with your feet shoulder-width apart, arms extended straight out to your sides at shoulder height.

2. **Circular Motion**: Slowly make small circles with your arms, gradually increasing the size of the circles.

3. **Direction**: After 10-15 circles, switch directions and repeat.

4. **Control**: Maintain a controlled motion, focusing on the shoulder joints.

<u>**Exercise 4 : Ankle Rolls**</u>

1. **Start Position**: Sit down on a chair and extend one leg out straight.

2. **Movement**: Rotate your foot at the ankle, making circular motions.

3. **Direction**: After 10-15 circles in one direction, switch and roll in the opposite direction.

4. **Switch**: Repeat the same process with the other foot.

<u>Part 2. Strength Exercises</u>

<u>**Exercise 5 : Chair Squats**</u>

1. **Start Position**: Stand in front of a sturdy chair with your feet shoulder-width apart.

2. **Movement**: Slowly lower your body as if to sit, bending at the knees and pushing your hips back.

3. **Pause**: Lightly touch the chair with your buttocks, but do not fully sit.

4. **Lift**: Engage your core and legs to return to a standing position.

5. **Modifications**: To make it easier, fully sit down then stand up. For more challenge, don't touch the chair at all.

6. **Repeat**: Do 10-15 repetitions.

Exercise 6 : Wall Push-Ups

1. **Start Position**: Face a wall, standing a little more than arm's length away, feet shoulder-width apart.

2. **Hands**: Place your hands flat against the wall at shoulder height and width.

3. **Movement**: Bend your elbows to bring your body closer to the wall, keeping your feet flat on the ground.

4. **Push**: Straighten your arms, pushing your body back to the starting position.

5. **Modifications**: Adjust your distance from the wall to increase or decrease difficulty.

6. **Repeat**: Perform 10-15 push-ups.

Exercise 7 : Toe Stands

1. **Start Position**: Stand behind a chair with your feet flat on the floor, holding onto the back of the chair for support.

2. **Movement**: Slowly raise your heels, standing on your toes.

3. **Hold**: Maintain the position for a few seconds.

4. **Lower**: Gently lower your heels back to the floor.

5. **Modifications**: To increase difficulty, try holding the position longer or performing the lift without support.

6. **Repeat**: Do 10-15 repetitions

This structure and content sample should serve as a robust foundation for creating a comprehensive, easy-to-follow exercise book for seniors. Ensure clarity and brevity in your instructions to make the routines accessible and the book an invaluable resource for senior health and well-being

Chapter Two : Balance Exercises

Exercise 1 Heel-to-Toe Walk

- **Instructions:**

1. Stand straight with your arms by your sides.

2. Step forward with one foot, placing the heel of your foot directly in front of the toes of the opposite foot.

3. Focus on a spot ahead of you to keep your balance.

4. Take a step with your other foot, bringing it in front of your opposite foot in a heel-to-toe motion.

5. Continue walking in a straight line for 15-20 steps.

- **Safety Tips:**

- Perform this exercise near a wall or a sturdy piece of furniture that you can hold onto if you feel unsteady.

- Wear supportive shoes to help maintain balance.

<u>**Exercise 2 Standing Leg Lifts**</u>

- **Instructions:**

1. Stand with your feet hip-width apart and hold onto a chair or counter for support.

2. Keeping your back straight and abdominal muscles engaged, slowly lift one leg to the side without tilting your torso.

3. Hold the position for a few seconds, then lower your leg back to the starting position.

4. Repeat 10-15 times on each leg.

- **Safety Tips:**

- Keep the movement controlled; do not swing your leg.

- Wear comfortable, supportive shoes to help with balance.

Chapter Three : Flexibility Exercises

Exercise 1 Seated Side Stretch

- **Instructions:**

1. Sit in a chair with your feet flat on the floor.

2. Extend your arms overhead, interlocking your fingers.

3. Gently lean to one side, feeling a stretch along your side. Hold for 15-30 seconds.

4. Return to the center and repeat on the other side.

Exercise 2 : Upper Body Stretch

- **Instructions:**

1. Stand up straight or sit in a chair without armrests.

2. Extend your arms out to the sides and then bring them behind your back.

3. Interlock your fingers and gently lift your arms, feeling the stretch across your chest and shoulders. Hold for 15-30 seconds.

Final Chapter The Cool Down Exercises

- **Gentle Walking in Place:**

1. Slowly walk in place, gradually lowering your pace to help your heart rate return to normal.

<u>Final stretches part 1- **Seated Forward Bend:**</u>

1. Sit on the edge of a chair with your feet flat on the ground.

2. Slowly bend forward at the hips, reaching towards your toes.

3. Hold this position for 15-30 seconds to stretch your lower back and hamstrings.

<u>Final stretch part 2-**Neck Stretch:**</u>

1. Sit or stand up straight.

2. Slowly tilt your head towards one shoulder until you feel a stretch.

3. Hold for 15-30 seconds, then repeat on the other.

Pointers Maintaining Your Routine

- **Tracking Your Progress:**

- Keep a journal or log of your exercises, including the type, duration, and how you felt.

- Note improvements in balance, flexibility, and strength over time.

- **Setting Realistic Goal:**

- Start with goals that are achievable and specific, such as "I will walk heel-to-toe for 10 steps without support by next month."

- Adjust your goals as you progress, always making sure they are realistic and motivating.

Final Authors note: I hope that you enjoyed the simplicity of this book and it helps you to regain your confidence and strengthen. Know that as you continue exercise you will continue improve your quality of life!

In Depth Analysis of Health Benefits: The Physical Health Perks of Exercise

The importance of exercise transcends the mere objective of achieving an ideal body weight or aesthetic physique. It embodies a multifaceted approach towards improving overall physical health and fortifying the body's resilience against diseases. This in-depth analysis aims to unravel the myriad physical health benefits attributed to regular exercise, based on current scientific understanding.

1. Cardiovascular Health Enhancement

At the core of exercise's health benefits is its capacity to significantly bolster cardiovascular health. Regular physical activity helps in regulating blood pressure, enhancing heart function, and improving blood circulation. Aerobic exercises, such as brisk walking, running, cycling, and swimming, have been shown to strengthen the heart muscle, thereby increasing its efficiency in pumping blood. This, in turn, reduces the resting heart rate and lowers blood pressure, mitigating the risk of heart diseases and stroke. Furthermore, exercise aids in increasing the levels of high-density lipoprotein (HDL), or "good" cholesterol, and reducing levels of low-density lipoprotein (LDL), or "bad" cholesterol, thus preventing arterial blockages.

2. Strengthening Musculoskeletal Health

Exercise is pivotal in enhancing musculoskeletal health. Weight-bearing exercises, including walking and resistance training, strengthen the bones, increase muscle mass, and improve joint flexibility. This is particularly vital in preventing osteoporosis - a condition characterized by weakened bones and increased fracture risk. Regular physical activity promotes the absorption of calcium and minerals into the bones, thereby making them denser and stronger. Moreover, by enhancing muscle strength and joint function, exercise also reduces the risk of musculoskeletal injuries.

3. Weight Management

Physical activity is a cornerstone in the management and prevention of obesity - a leading risk factor for numerous chronic diseases. Exercise expends energy, thereby helping in burning calories and reducing body fat. By increasing the metabolic rate, it not only aids in weight loss but also in maintaining weight loss over time. Furthermore, muscle mass is maintained or increased through exercise, which in itself burns more calories than fat, thus favoring a more favorable body composition.

4. Diabetes Control

Regular exercise plays a crucial role in regulating blood sugar levels and improving insulin sensitivity, making it a key factor in the management and prevention of Type 2 diabetes. By facilitating the muscle's uptake of glucose, exercise can help in lowering blood sugar levels, thereby reducing the need for insulin. This not only helps in managing diabetes among those who have been diagnosed but also reduces the risk of developing the condition.

5. Enhancing Respiratory and Pulmonary Function

Exercise also has significant benefits for the respiratory system. It increases lung capacity and efficiency in oxygen exchange, thereby improving endurance and reducing fatigue. Regular physical activity can help in preventing or managing chronic respiratory diseases such as chronic obstructive pulmonary disease (COPD) and asthma by enhancing the strength of respiratory muscles.

6. Immune System Boost

Engaging in regular physical activity has been linked to a strengthened immune system. Exercise promotes the circulation of immune cells, making it easier for the body to detect and combat infections. While intense physical activity can temporarily suppress the immune system, moderate exercise strengthens it by improving vaccination responses, reducing inflammation, and enhancing the body's ability to prevent and recover from infections.

7. Reduction in Cancer Risk

Evidence indicates that regular exercise is associated with a lowered risk of developing certain types of cancer, notably breast, colon, and lung cancer. While the mechanisms underlying this protective effect are still being explored, exercise is known to reduce inflammation, improve immune function, and decrease levels of certain hormones that can fuel cancer growth.

Conclusion

The physical health benefits of exercise are profound and encompass more than just improved aesthetics. From cardiovascular health to weight management, diabetes control, and cancer risk reduction, the positive implications of regular physical activity are undeniable. It is a cornerstone of preventive medicine and a prescription for a healthier, more vibrant life. As research continues to evolve, it further underscores the necessity of incorporating exercise into our daily routines for optimal physical health.

Certainly! Weight-bearing exercises are crucial for building and maintaining bone density as well as muscle strength. By incorporating these types of exercises into your routine, you can significantly improve your overall health and reduce the risk of osteoporosis and other bone-related conditions. Here are some specific weight-bearing exercises that are particularly effective in strengthening bones and muscles:

1. **Walking and Hiking**: Simple yet effective. Walking, especially brisk walking, and hiking on various terrains can help strengthen the muscles in your legs and spine, and stimulate bone growth due to the impact involved.

2. **Strength Training**: This includes using free weights, weight machines, or resistance bands. Exercises like squats, lunges, deadlifts, and bench presses target multiple muscle groups and bones, promoting bone growth and muscular strength.

Title: Unveiling the Power of Home-Based Strength Training: A Comprehensive Guide

Introduction

In recent times, the advent of home workouts has revolutionized how we approach fitness, breaking the myth that effective strength training is confined to the gym. This comprehensive guide will unveil the multifaceted benefits of strength training and shed light on the best practices for engaging in these exercises safely and effectively from the comfort of your home.

The Multifold Benefits of Strength Training

1. Enhanced Muscular and Bone Health

Strength training, also known as resistance training, plays a pivotal role in augmenting muscle mass and enhancing bone density. This form of exercise is instrumental in counteracting the muscle loss that accompanies aging and in preventing osteoporosis, thereby paving the way for a robust and resilient body.

2. Boosted Metabolic Rate

Regular strength training elevates your resting metabolic rate, meaning your body burns calories more efficiently even when you're not working out. This metabolic boost is a cornerstone for weight management and for preventing obesity-related health conditions.

3. Improved Functional Fitness

The strength garnered from regular training transcends aesthetic appeal, significantly enhancing your ability to perform daily tasks with ease. From lifting groceries to climbing stairs, the functional fitness derived from strength training is invaluable.

4. Augmentation of Mental Health

Beyond the physical benefits, strength training has been shown to alleviate symptoms of depression and anxiety, enhance cognitive function, and boost overall mood. This is attributed to the endorphin release, often referred to as the "runner's high," which is also present during high-intensity strength workouts.

Best Practices for Home-Based Strength Training

1. Start with the Basics

Embarking on a strength training journey doesn't require fancy equipment. Bodyweight exercises like push-ups, squats, and lunges are foundational movements that effectively build strength. As you progress, incorporating resistance bands or handheld weights can add variety and intensity to your routines.

2. Ensure Proper Form and Technique

The cornerstone of safe strength training is maintaining proper form. Incorrect posture or technique can lead to injury, hampering your fitness journey. Online tutorials, fitness apps, or virtual personal training sessions can be invaluable resources for learning and refining your technique.

3. Gradually Increase Intensity

Adherence to the principle of progressive overload — gradually increasing the weight, frequency, or number of repetitions in your strength training routine — is key to continuous improvement. This approach promotes muscle growth and endurance without overwhelming your body.

4. Balance Your Routine

A well-rounded strength training program involves working all major muscle groups to ensure balanced muscle development and prevent overuse injuries. Incorporating rest days is equally important to allow your muscles to recover and grow.

5. Listen to Your Body

Adopting a mindful approach to training by listening to your body's signals is paramount. Rest when needed and don't push through pain. Understanding the difference between the discomfort associated with muscle fatigue and the pain indicative of injury is critical for safe training.

Conclusion

Strength training from home is a viable and effective way to enhance your physical and mental well-being. By embracing the principles of progression, balance, and mindfulness, you can harness the benefits of strength training, achieving a stronger, healthier body without stepping foot in a gym. Remember, consistency is key; dedication to your home workout routine will yield remarkable results over time. Begin your strength training journey today and unlock the door to a healthier, more vibrant you.

3. **Jogging/Running**:

More high-impact than walking, jogging and running exert more force on the bones, helping to stimulate bone growth. It's particularly good for the legs and hips.

4. **Stair Climbing**:

Climbing stairs is a powerful weight-bearing activity that engages several muscle groups in your lower body while also putting pressure on your bones to stimulate growth.

5. **Dancing**:

Fast-paced dancing styles that involve jumping and hopping are excellent for bone health. They not only work on your lower body but can also be a full-body workout.

6. **Yoga and Pilates**:

Although they are low-impact, some poses and movements specifically target bone and muscle strength, balance, and flexibility. Poses like the Warrior series, Tree Pose, and Planks are beneficial.

7. **Jumping Rope**:

This high-impact exercise is excellent for increasing bone density in the legs and hips. It also significantly improves cardiovascular health and endurance.

8. **Tennis or Other Racket Sports**:

These sports require quick, forceful movements and changes of direction that stress the bones in a beneficial way, particularly in the arms and legs.

9. **Elliptical Training and Aerobics**:

Low-impact aerobic exercises can also be effective, especially for those who may not be able to tolerate high-impact activities. They help improve cardiovascular health and maintain bone density.

In addition to these exercises, incorporating balance and flexibility exercises can help reduce the risk of falls, leading to fractures, especially in older adults. It's also important to note that consistency and gradually increasing the intensity of these activities can yield the best results for bone and muscle health.

As with starting any new exercise regimen, it's wise to consult with a healthcare provider or a fitness professional, especially if you have existing health concerns, to design a program that's tailored to your specific needs and goals.

Certainly! Below is a detailed workout schedule focused on weight-bearing exercises for bone and muscle strengthening.

This routine is designed to be performed over a week, incorporating rest days to allow for recovery. Adjust the weights used according to your fitness level and aim to progressively increase the weights or resistance as you get stronger.

Day 1: Lower Body & Core

- **Warm-up**: 10 minutes of brisk walking or cycling

- **Squats**: 3 sets of 12 reps

- **Lunges**: 3 sets of 10 reps per leg

- **Deadlifts**: 3 sets of 10 reps

- **Leg Press**: 3 sets of 12 reps

- **Calf Raises**: 3 sets of 15 reps

- **Plank**: 3 sets of 30-60 seconds

- **Side Plank**: 3 sets of 30 seconds per side

- **Cooldown**: Stretching focusing on legs and core, 10 minutes

Day 2: Upper Body

- **Warm-up**: 10 minutes of jump rope or arm circles

- **Push-ups**: 3 sets of 12 reps

- **Pull-ups or Lat Pull-downs**: 3 sets of 10 reps

- **Dumbbell Bench Press**: 3 sets of 12 reps

- **Dumbbell Rows**: 3 sets of 12 reps per arm

- **Shoulder Press**: 3 sets of 12 reps

- **Tricep Dips**: 3 sets of 10 reps

- **Bicep Curls**: 3 sets of 12 reps per arm

- **Cooldown**: Stretching focusing on upper body, 10 minutes

Day 3: Rest or Light Cardio

- **Activities**: Walking, yoga, or swimming for 20-30 minutes

Day 4: Cardio & Core

- **Warm-up**: 5 minutes of dynamic stretching

- **Interval Running or Cycling**: 20 minutes (1-minute sprint followed by 2 minutes of light pace)

- **Russian Twists**: 3 sets of 15 reps per side

- **Leg Raises**: 3 sets of 12 reps

- **Mountain Climbers**: 3 sets of 30 seconds

- **Cooldown**: Stretching, focusing on flexibility and core, 10 minutes

Day 5: Compound Movements

- **Warm-up**: 10 minutes of brisk walking or cycling

- **Deadlifts**: 4 sets of 8 reps

- **Bench Press**: 4 sets of 8 reps

- **Squats**: 4 sets of 8 reps

- **Pull-ups or Lat Pull-downs**: 4 sets of 10 reps

- **Dumbbell Lunges**: 3 sets of 10 reps per leg

- **Cooldown**: Full body stretching, 10 minutes

Day 6: Rest or Active Recovery

- **Activities**: Gentle cycling, walking, foam rolling, or yoga

Day 7: Mix Day or Rest

- **Option 1 (Mix Day)**: Mix of cardio (30 minutes of moderate-intensity) and full body light weight training or bodyweight exercises (1 set of 15 reps)

- **Option 2 (Rest)**: Complete rest or gentle stretching/yoga

Notes:

- Ensure to hydrate properly and consume a balanced diet rich in protein, vitamins, and minerals to support recovery and bone health.

- Listen to your body and adjust the intensity or take extra rest days as needed.

This schedule can be repeated, with incremental increases in intensity or weights to continue building bone density and muscle strength over time.

For people with joint issues, engaging in exercises that promote flexibility, strength, and cardiovascular health while minimizing stress on the joints is crucial. Here's a detailed list of alternative exercises designed to be gentle on the joints:

1. **Swimming and Water Aerobics**:

Water provides buoyancy that supports the body, reducing stress on the joints. The resistance of water also offers a great way to strengthen muscles. Swimming laps or participating in water aerobics classes can improve heart health, flexibility, and muscle strength.

2. **Walking**:

Walking, especially on flat surfaces, can be a low-impact cardiovascular exercise. Wearing supportive shoes can help reduce the stress on knee and hip joints. For added benefits, walking in shallow water in a pool can also reduce joint strain.

3. **Cycling**:

Using a stationary bike or cycling outdoors on a regular bike is excellent for the knees and hips because it keeps them moving through a range of motion with minimal impact. Adjusting the seat height correctly ensures that the knees do not suffer from overextension.

4. **Elliptical Training**:

An elliptical machine provides a good cardiovascular workout similar to jogging but with significantly less stress on the joints. The smooth, gliding motions allow for heart rate elevation without the harsh impact of other activities.

5. **Yoga**:

Yoga helps improve flexibility, strength, and balance. Certain poses are gentle on the joints and can be modified to suit individual needs. The emphasis on breathing and mindfulness also contributes to reducing stress and improving overall well-being.

Modifying yoga poses for joint issues is crucial for ensuring practice sustainability and preventing injury. Here is how you can adapt some common yoga poses to be more joint-friendly:

1. **For Knee Issues**

- **Chair Pose** Instead of going into a deep squat, decrease the bend in your knees to reduce pressure on them. Use a chair for support if needed.

- **Warrior Poses** Shorten your stance to lessen the strain on your knee joints. Ensure your knee does not extend past your ankle in the bent-leg positions.

2. **For Wrist Issues**

- **Downward-Facing Dog** Use foam wedges under your hands to decrease the angle of wrist extension, or perform the pose on your forearms to completely avoid wrist extension.

- **Plank Pose**: Similar to Downward-Facing Dog, you can perform the plank on your forearms to relieve pressure off your wrists.

3. **For Shoulder Issues**

Instead of the full pose, bring your knees down to the floor, reducing the amount of body weight your shoulders have to bear.

- **Cow Face Pose** Use a strap between your hands if you cannot comfortably clasp your hands together behind your back, to avoid overstretching and stressing the shoulder joints.

4. **For Ankle Issues**

- **Tree Pose** Instead of placing the foot on the inner thigh or calf, rest it on the ankle of the standing leg with the toes on the floor for balance and minimal ankle strain.

- **Standing Forward Fold** Bend your knees slightly to alleviate tension in the ankles and hamstrings.

5. **For Neck Issues**

- **Rabbit Pose** Keep the neck in a neutral position rather than forcing it into flexion. Support the head with your hands or a cushion.

- **Shoulder Stand** Use multiple folded blankets under your shoulders to elevate the neck and shoulders off the floor, ensuring no direct pressure is on the neck.

General Tips

- **Use Props**: Incorporate yoga blocks, straps, bolsters, and blankets to find comfortable positions and maintain proper alignment.

- **Don't Push Through Pain**: Listen to your body and avoid any movement that causes pain.

- **Consult a Professional**: Work with a yoga teacher experienced in therapeutic yoga or a physical therapist knowledgeable in yoga to customize your practice.

Creating a yoga practice that accommodates joint issues involves mindful adjustments and recognizing your body's limits. Regularly incorporating these modifications can help you enjoy the benefits of yoga with less risk of exacerbating joint pain or injuries.

Yes, modifying yoga poses for individuals with joint issues is essential for ensuring a safe and effective practice. Here are some suggestions for modifications of common yoga poses to help accommodate joint issues:

1. **Downward-Facing Dog**

   - **Modification**: Use yoga blocks under your hands if you have wrist issues. This decreases the angle and pressure on your wrists. Alternatively, practice the dolphin pose, which uses forearms instead of hands, to relieve pressure on the wrists.

2. **Warrior II**

- **Modification**: For those with knee issues, ensure the bent knee does not extend past the toes to prevent additional strain. You can also decrease the depth of the lunge to reduce pressure on the knees.

3. **Chair Pose**

- **Modification**: To ease pressure on the knees, avoid bending too deeply. Keep the pose more upright and use a wall for support if necessary.

4. **Pigeon Pose**

- **Modification**: For those with hip or knee concerns, perform a modified pigeon on your back by crossing one ankle over the opposite knee and gently pulling the thigh towards your chest. This reduces pressure on the joints.

5. **Triangle Pose**

   - **Modification**: Use a yoga block under your lower hand if you cannot comfortably reach the floor. This helps maintain alignment without overstretching or stressing the joints.

6. **Cobra Pose**

   - **Modification**: If you have back issues, practice a gentle version by keeping your elbows bent and forearms on the ground, lifting your chest only as far as comfortable. This is known as Sphinx Pose.

7. **Child's Pose**

- **Modification**: If you have knee issues, place a folded blanket between your thighs and calves or under your buttocks for added support and to lessen the bend of the knees.

8. **Tree Pose**

- **Modification**: For individuals with ankle or balance issues, perform the pose with your back against a wall for support, or keep the toes of your lifted foot on the ground and rest the heel against the ankle of the standing leg.

When practicing yoga with joint issues, the focus should be on maintaining a balance between flexibility and stability, ensuring that you do not overextend or place undue pressure on affected joints. Listening to your body and using props such as blocks, straps, and blankets can also help achieve a safe and beneficial practice. Always consult with a healthcare professional or a specialized yoga instructor before starting or modifying your practice, especially if you have significant joint concerns.

Practicing yoga with wrist pain requires a mindful approach to avoid aggravating the condition. Here are several strategies and modifications to help you continue practicing yoga safely:

1. **Wrist Warm-ups:**

Begin your practice with gentle wrist stretches and rotations to increase blood flow and flexibility in the wrist area.

2. **Weight Distribution:**

Be conscious of how you distribute your weight in poses that involve the hands. Spread your fingers wide and press down through the base of your fingers to decrease pressure on your wrists.

3. **Use Props:**

Utilize props such as yoga blocks or wedges under your hands in poses like Downward Dog, Plank, or Crow to reduce the angle and pressure on your wrists. This modification helps align the wrists in a more neutral position.

4. **Forearm Modifications:**

Substitute wrist-loading poses with forearm variations. For example, practice Dolphin Pose instead of Downward Facing Dog, or Forearm Plank instead of High Plank. This approach significantly reduces wrist strain.

5. **Strengthen and Stretch:**

Incorporate exercises that strengthen the muscles around your wrists and arms, as well as stretching exercises to improve flexibility. This can help support your joints better and potentially reduce pain over time.

6. **Avoid or Modify Certain Poses:**

Be careful with poses that place a lot of stress on your wrists. If a specific pose causes discomfort, either modify it with the help of props or skip it entirely. Listening to your body is key.

7. **Use a Soft Surface:**

Practicing on a softer surface or folding your yoga mat for extra padding under your hands can reduce the strain on your wrists.

8. **Limit Repetitive Strain:**

Pay attention to the frequency of poses that strain your wrists. Balance your practice with poses that don't involve wrist pressure.

9. **Mindful Transitions:**

Be mindful of how you transition between poses, especially those that require placing your hands on the floor. Move slowly and with intention to avoid sudden pressure on your wrists.

10. **Consult a Professional:**

If your wrist pain persists, consider consulting a healthcare professional or a physical therapist specialized in yoga or sports injuries. They can provide personalized advice and possibly identify the root cause of your pain.

Incorporating wrist-strengthening exercises into your yoga practice is a great idea, especially to support poses that place stress on your wrists and to prevent injuries. Here are some tips and exercises you can easily integrate into your yoga routine:

1. **Warm-Up Your Wrists:**

Begin your practice with gentle wrist stretches to increase blood flow and flexibility. Circle your wrists in both directions, flex and extend the wrist, and do side-to-side movements.

2. **Focus on Alignment:**

In any weight-bearing poses like Downward Dog, Plank, or Crow Pose, ensure proper hand placement and alignment. Spread your fingers wide, press down through the base of each finger, and slightly rotate your forearms outward to engage and protect the wrists.

3. **Wrist Strengthening Exercises:**

   - **Wrist Curls:** You can do these with a lightweight or no weight at all. Extend your arms in front of you with palms facing up, and curl the wrists toward your body.

   - **Reverse Wrist Curls:** Similar to wrist curls, but with palms facing down. This helps strengthen the extensor muscles.

   - **Tiger Claws:** Extend your arms in front of you with palms facing down. Make a fist, then open your hand, spreading your fingers as wide as possible. Repeat several times to improve strength and flexibility.

4. **Practice Weight-Bearing Poses Gradually:**

Gradually increase the time you spend in poses that put pressure on your wrists. Begin with shorter intervals and incrementally add time as your wrists become stronger.

5. **Use Props:**

Use props to alleviate pressure on your wrists. For example, a folded blanket under the heels of your hands in Downward Dog or wrist wedges can change the angle of the wrist and reduce strain.

6. **Incorporate Non-Weight Bearing Poses:**

Ensure your practice includes a balance of poses that do not stress the wrists. These poses give your wrists time to rest and recover while you focus on other aspects of your practice.

7. **Strengthen the Surrounding Areas:**

Strengthening your shoulders, arms, and core can also help, as these muscles support your body in various poses and reduce the load on your wrists.

8. **Listen to Your Body:**

Pay attention to any signs of discomfort or strain in your wrists. If you feel pain, ease off and consider modifying the pose or using props to support your practice.

Incorporating these tips into your yoga practice can help you build stronger wrists, improve your poses, and minimize the risk of injury. Remember, consistency is key, so make wrist health a regular part of your yoga routine.

Remember, yoga is about connecting with your body in a compassionate way. Never force yourself into pain, and always prioritize your well-being over achieving a particular pose. With these modifications and a mindful approach, you can continue to enjoy the benefits of yoga without exacerbating wrist pain.

6. **Tai Chi**:

This martial art involves slow, controlled movements and deep breathing. It is excellent for balance, flexibility, and mental focus. Tai Chi is particularly beneficial for those with arthritis as it helps increase range of motion and decrease pain.

7. **Pilates**:

Pilates focuses on core strength, flexibility, and overall body awareness. Using mats or specialized equipment like reformers, Pilates exercises can be adjusted to avoid putting unnecessary strain on joints.

Pilates is a form of low-impact exercise that aims to strengthen muscles while improving postural alignment and flexibility. It was created by Joseph Pilates in the early 20th century and was initially used as a rehabilitation technique for wounded soldiers during World War I. Pilates focuses on precision movements coming from the center of the body, which is often referred to as the "powerhouse" and includes the abdominal muscles, lower back, hips, and buttocks.

There are two main types of Pilates:

1. **Mat Pilates:**

This is the most accessible form, requiring only a mat and your body. It focuses on performing controlled movements in various positions to strengthen the body with gravity as the main resistance.

2. **Reformer Pilates:**

This involves a machine called a Reformer, which looks like a bed frame with a sliding carriage and adjustable springs to regulate tension and resistance. Cables, bars, straps, and pulleys allow exercises to be performed in a variety of positions, increasing effectiveness and adding versatility.

Pilates exercises are designed to align, stretch, and strengthen the body without adding bulk. This is why it is a popular choice among dancers and athletes for cross-training. It emphasizes breath, alignment, balance, strength, and flexibility. With its focus on mindful movement, Pilates has also been noted to have benefits on mental health, reducing stress, and improving concentration and wellbeing.

Anyone, from beginners to advanced practitioners, can do Pilates. It offers a range of difficulty levels, from fundamental movements to advanced sequences, making it accessible and challenging for people at any stage of fitness. Regular Pilates practice can contribute to improving posture, muscle tone, balance, and joint mobility, as well as relieve stress and tension.

Certainly! Here are five beginner-friendly Pilates exercises that are ideal for starting your Pilates journey. These exercises focus on core strength, flexibility, and control, which are central to Pilates principles. Ensure that you perform each exercise with careful attention to form and breath control.

1. **The Hundred**

- Lie on your back with your knees bent into your chest and feet lifted into a tabletop position.

- Lift your head, neck, and shoulders off the mat, extending your arms by your sides.

- Vigorously pump your arms up and down in a small range of motion, inhaling for five arm pumps and exhaling for five pumps.

- Aim for 100 pumps.

2. **Pelvic Curl**

- Lie on your back with your knees bent and feet flat on the floor, hip-distance apart.

- Inhale to prepare, then exhale as you slowly curl your spine off the floor, starting from your tailbone and moving up through your spine until your body forms a straight line from shoulders to knees.

- Inhale at the top, then exhale as you slowly lower your spine back down to the mat, one vertebra at a time.

3. **Single Leg Circles**

- Lie on your back with one leg extended towards the ceiling and the other flat on the mat. Keep your arms by your sides and palms pressing down.

- Circle the raised leg across your body, then down around and back to the center in a controlled manner. Keep your hips still and the rest of your body grounded.

- Do 5 circles in each direction, then switch legs.

4. **Spine Stretch**

- Sit up tall with your legs extended in front of you, wider than hip-distance apart, feet flexed.

- Inhale to prepare, then exhale as you reach your arms forward and curve your spine into a "C" shape, stretching forward from your waist.

- Hold for a breath, then slowly stack your spine back up to sitting.

5. **Swan Prep**

- Lie on your stomach with your hands under your shoulders and elbows close to your body.

- Engage your abdominal muscles to protect your lower back. Inhale as you gently extend your spine to lift your head and chest off the floor, using your back muscles, not your hands.

- Exhale as you lower back down.

These exercises provide a solid foundation in the core principles of Pilates, such as breathing, concentration, control, and precision. Always pay close attention to your body, ensuring that you do not strain or rush the movements. Starting with these basics can help you build a strong foundation and eventually progress to more advanced exercises.

8. **Resistance Training with Bands or Light Weights**: Resistance exercises increase muscle strength without needing to lift heavy weights. Using resistance bands or light dumbbells for exercises can help protect joint health while still building strength. Focus on controlled movements and proper form.

Resistance training with bands or light weights can both be highly effective for building strength, improving muscle tone, and enhancing overall fitness. Each method comes with its unique benefits and considerations. Here's a detailed comparison to help you decide which might be best for your fitness goals.

Resistance Bands

Pros:

- **Versatility and Portability:**

Resistance bands are lightweight, portable, and can be used virtually anywhere. They are ideal for home workouts, traveling, or outdoor exercises.

- **Progressive Resistance:**

As the band stretches, the resistance increases, offering a unique resistance profile that is different from free weights. This can lead to increased muscle activation throughout the range of motion.

- **Cost-Effective:**

Generally, bands are less expensive than a set of weights and can provide a wide range of resistance levels from light to very heavy.

- **Joint-Friendly:**

The elastic nature of bands can be gentler on the joints, making them suitable for rehabilitation or those with joint concerns.

Cons:

- **Durability Issues:** Over time, bands can wear out, lose elasticity, or even snap, posing a risk of injury.

- **Limited Maximal Resistance:**

Bands have a finite length they can stretch, which may limit the maximal resistance they can provide, potentially limiting strength gains in more advanced exercisers.

- **Difficulty Quantifying Progress:**

With bands, it's harder to measure progress since the resistance is not as clearly quantifiable as lifting a certain weight.

Light Weights

Pros:

- **Simplicity:**

Light weights (dumbbells, kettlebells) are straightforward to use and make it easy to understand and track progression by moving up in weight.

- **Stability and Control:**

Weights offer a consistent resistance that can help with developing balance and muscle coordination, as the lifter must control the weight through the entire range of motion.

- **Variety:**

A vast array of exercises can be performed with light weights, effectively targeting every major muscle group with different movements.

- **Increased Bone Density:**

Using weights can help increase bone density and strength, reducing the risk of osteoporosis.

Cons:

- **Space and Cost:**

A full set of weights can be more expensive and requires more space for storage than a set of resistance bands.

- **Risk of Injury:**

Incorrect form or using excessively heavy weights can lead to injuries. Proper technique and gradual progression are essential.

- **Portability:**

Weights are not as portable as bands, making them less convenient for those who travel frequently or lack space.

Conclusion

The choice between resistance bands and light weights depends on your specific goals, preferences, availability of equipment, and any physical considerations. For beginners, those with limited space, or people who travel often, resistance bands are a great choice. For those focusing on building muscle mass, improving bone density, or who enjoy weightlifting workouts, light weights might be more beneficial. Many individuals find incorporating both into their fitness routine offers the best of both worlds, providing variety and comprehensive benefits.

9. ** Isometric Exercises**:

These exercises involve tightening muscles without moving the joints, making them an excellent option for individuals with joint pain. They help in maintaining muscle strength without adding pressure to the joints.

Isometric exercises are a form of resistance training in which the joint angle and muscle length do not change during contraction. Unlike dynamic exercises, where muscles lengthen and shorten through movements, isometric exercises involve exerting force against a stationary object or holding a position without movement. This type of exercise can be very efficient for building strength, endurance, and stability in muscles without putting too much strain on the joints. They are particularly beneficial for rehabilitation, improving posture, and enhancing static muscle strength.

Here are some examples of isometric exercises:

1. **Plank**:

Involves holding your body in a straight line from head to heels, supported by your forearms and toes.

2. **Wall Sit**:

Leaning against a wall, slide down until your knees are at a 90-degree angle, and hold this position.

3. **Bridge Hold**:

Lie on your back with knees bent, feet flat on the floor, then lift your hips towards the ceiling and hold.

4. **Isometric Push-up Hold**:

Start in a push-up position and lower yourself halfway, then hold.

5. **Squat Hold**:

Lower into a squat position and hold it without moving up or down.

6. **Isometric Bicep Hold**:

Hold a dumbbell or a resistance band in front of you with your elbow bent at 90 degrees, keeping the muscle contracted without movement.

7. **L-Sit**:

Sit on the floor with your legs straight in front of you, place your hands beside your hips, then lift your body off the ground, keeping your legs straight.

Benefits of isometric exercises include:

- **Improved Muscle Strength**: They can target specific muscle groups and improve overall muscle strength.

- **Increased Muscle Endurance**: Holding positions for longer periods can increase muscle stamina.

- **Enhanced Stability and Balance**: By engaging and strengthening the core muscles, isometric exercises can improve your balance and posture.

- **Injury Recovery and Prevention**: Since they put less strain on joints and tendons, isometric exercises are often used in physical therapy and rehabilitation.

- **Accessibility**: They can be performed anywhere, without the need for equipment or large spaces.

To get the most out of isometric exercises, it's important to breathe properly, maintain good form, and gradually increase hold times as your strength and endurance improve. Always consult with a fitness professional or a medical advisor to ensure these exercises are suitable for your specific health and fitness levels, especially if you have existing health conditions or injuries.

10. ** Chair Exercises**: For those with severe joint issues, chair exercises—whether it's upper body movements, leg raises, or light resistance exercises—can be performed while sitting down, reducing the risk of falls and joint strain.

Chair exercises are a fantastic way to stay active and improve your fitness, especially for those who have limited mobility, are new to exercise, or spend a lot of time sitting at a desk. They can enhance flexibility, strength, and cardiovascular health. Here's a quick guide to some effective chair exercises:

1. Seated Marches

- **How to:** Sit up straight on the edge of the chair with feet flat on the ground. March your legs up and down one at a time, lifting your knees as high as possible.

- **Benefits:** Increases heart rate, strengthens the legs.

2. Chair Squats

- **How to:** Stand in front of a chair with feet hip-width apart. Slowly lower yourself down until your backside touches the chair, then stand back up.

- **Benefits:** Strengthens buttocks, thighs, and improves balance.

3. Seated Leg Lifts

- **How to:** Sit on the edge of the chair with legs extended straight out. Lift one leg at a time as high as possible, keeping the knee straight.

- **Benefits:** Strengthens the quadriceps.

4. Arm Circles

- **How to:** Sit or stand and extend your arms straight out to the sides at shoulder height. Circle your arms forward for a set time, then reverse the direction.

- **Benefits:** Tones and strengthens shoulders.

5. Chair Yoga Poses

- **Example:** Cat-Cow Stretch

  - **How to:** Sit on the edge of the chair with feet flat. Place hands on knees. As you inhale, arch your back and look upward (Cow), as you exhale, round your back and tuck your chin (Cat).

  - **Benefits:** Increases flexibility and relieves tension in the spine.

6. Seated Russian Twists

- **How to:** Sit on the edge of the chair, lean back slightly, keeping the spine straight. Clasp your hands in front of you and twist your torso to the right, then to the left.

- **Benefits:** Strengthens core, obliques.

Tips for Chair Exercises:

- **Warm-Up:** Start with light stretching or simple movements to get the blood flowing.

- **Posture:** Keep your back straight and abdominals engaged during exercises.

- **Breathing:** Don't hold your breath. Inhale and exhale fully during movements.

- **Frequency:** Aim for at least 30 minutes of moderate-intensity exercise per day, as recommended by health organizations. Chair exercises can be broken into shorter segments throughout the day if needed.

These exercises are versatile and can be modified to suit different fitness levels. They're also especially beneficial for older adults, those recovering from injury, or individuals with disabilities. Always consult with a healthcare provider before starting any new exercise program, especially if you have existing health concerns.

Certainly! Chair exercises are a great option for seniors looking to maintain or improve their strength, flexibility, and circulation while minimizing the risk of injury. Here are some additional chair exercises geared toward seniors:

1. **Leg Lifts**

- Sit upright with your feet flat on the floor.

- Straighten one leg at a time and lift it to a comfortable height.

- Hold for a few seconds, then slowly lower it.

- Repeat with the other leg.

- Aim for 10-15 repetitions per leg.

2. **Seated Marching**

- Sit upright and march your legs up and down in place.

- Lift your knees as high as comfortable.

- Continue for 30 seconds to 1 minute.

3. **Arm Circles**

- Sit with your arms extended by your sides, parallel to the floor.

- Make small circles with your arms, gradually increasing the size of the circles.

- After 30 seconds, reverse the direction.

- Perform for 1-2 minutes.

4. **Side Bends**

- Sit upright with your feet flat and spread apart.

- Place one hand behind your head and the other arm outstretched to the side.

- Bend to the side, moving the outstretched arm towards the floor.

- Return to the starting position and repeat on the other side.

- Do 8-10 repetitions per side.

5. **Seated Cat-Cow Stretch**

- Place your hands on your knees.

- Inhale, arch your back and look up towards the ceiling (Cow position).

- Exhale, round your spine while tucking your chin to your chest (Cat position).

- Alternate between these two positions for 8-10 cycles.

6. **Ankle Circles**

- Lift one foot off the floor.

- Rotating at the ankle, draw circles in the air with your toes.

- Do 10 circles in one direction, then switch directions.

- Repeat with the other foot.

7. **Chair Stand (for strength and balance)**

- Sit in a chair with your feet flat on the floor, shoulder-width apart.

- Extend your arms parallel to the floor.

- Lean forward slightly and stand up, using your leg muscles.

- Slowly lower yourself back down to the sitting position.

- Aim for 8-10 repetitions.

8. **Wrist Flex and Extend**

- Extend one arm out with your palm facing down.

- Gently pull the fingers back with the other hand for a stretch.

- Hold for a few seconds, then point the fingers down and stretch.

- Repeat on the other arm.

Incorporating chair exercises into your daily routine is a fantastic way to stay active, especially if you spend a lot of time sitting for work or if you're looking for low-impact options. Here are some tips to effectively integrate these exercises into your day:

1. **Set Regular Reminders**: Use your phone or computer to set reminders to take short exercise breaks throughout the day. Every hour, try to spend 5-10 minutes doing a selection of chair exercises.

2. **Create a Routine**: Structure a routine that combines various exercises to target different parts of the body. Include stretches, muscle-strengthening exercises, and aerobic movements. Doing the same routine can help form a habit.

3. **Use What You Have**: You don't necessarily need special equipment. For some exercises, the chair and your body weight are enough. For added resistance, you can use water bottles, books, or resistance bands.

4. **Incorporate Exercises into Daily Tasks**: Integrate exercises into activities you're already doing. For example, try leg lifts or ankle circles while reading emails or seated marches when on a call.

5. **Stay Consistent**: Consistency is key. It might be helpful to exercise at the same time each day to establish a routine.

6. **Increase Difficulty Gradually**: As you get more comfortable with the exercises, start increasing the intensity. This could mean adding more repetitions, holding positions longer, or incorporating weights.

7. **Track Your Progress**: Keep a journal or use an app to track the exercises you're doing, how often, and any progress you notice. This is motivating and helps you to adjust your routine as needed.

8. **Stay Safe**: Choose a sturdy chair without wheels, and ensure it's on a stable surface to prevent slipping or tipping. Listen to your body, and avoid movements that cause pain.

9. **Mix It Up**: To prevent boredom and target different muscle groups, vary your exercises. There are many resources online for chair-based exercises offering variety and challenges.

10. **Double Up on Activities**: Consider pairing your exercise routine with something enjoyable, like watching your favorite TV show, listening to a podcast, or catching up on audiobooks. This can make the time more enjoyable and something you look forward to.

11. **Engage with a Community**: Join a group or find friends who are also interested in staying active. Sharing routines, progress, and challenges can be motivating.

Incorporating chair exercises into your daily routine doesn't have to be daunting. By setting small, achievable goals and gradually integrating these exercises into your daily activities, you can improve your health, flexibility, and overall well-being with minimal disruption to your day.

These exercises are designed to be safe and effective for most seniors, but it's always recommended to consult with a healthcare provider before starting any new exercise regime, especially if you have any health concerns or conditions.

When trying these exercises, it's essential to listen to your body and avoid movements that cause pain. Consulting with a physical therapist or exercise specialist who can tailor a program to fit your specific health and fitness needs is also beneficial. Starting slowly and gradually increasing the duration and intensity of the workouts as your strength and flexibility improve will yield the best outcomes.

Exercising regularly has numerous mental health benefits, including:

1. **Reduced Symptoms of Depression and Anxiety**: Engaging in regular physical activity is believed to increase the production of endorphins, commonly known as the

body's "feel-good" neurotransmitters. This can help reduce feelings of depression, anxiety, and stress by improving your mood and distracting you from worries.

2. **Enhanced Mood**: Regular exercise can improve your mood and decrease feelings of depression, anxiety, and stress. The chemical changes in the brain can moderate the brain's reaction to stress, making you feel more relaxed and happier.

3. **Improved Sleep**: Exercise can help you fall asleep faster and deepen your sleep. The energy depletion that occurs during exercise stimulates recuperative processes during sleep, and the increase in body temperature may also help to improve sleep quality.

4. **Increased Self-Esteem and Confidence**: Regular physical activity can boost your self-esteem and confidence. By meeting exercise goals or challenges, even small ones, you can feel a sense of achievement.

5. **Cognitive Benefits**: Exercise can improve brain function. It increases heart rate, which pumps more oxygen to the brain. It can also promote the growth of new brain cells and prevent age-related decline.

6. **Better Resilience**: Engaging in regular physical activity can help you develop resilience to stress factors by mimicking stress on the body (physical stress of exercising) and helping the body practice dealing with stress.

7. **Greater Creativity and Productivity**: Exercise can also boost creativity and productivity. It helps to clear the mind, improves decision-making capabilities, and boosts your energy levels, which can lead to increased productivity at work or school.

By integrating regular exercise into your lifestyle, you can experience a wide range of mental health benefits that contribute to overall wellbeing.

Staying motivated to exercise regularly, especially for its mental health benefits, involves combining both internal and external strategies. Here are some tips to help keep you on track:

1. **Set Clear, Achievable Goals**: Start with simple goals and then progress to longer-range goals. Remember to make them SMART (Specific, Measurable, Achievable, Relevant, and Time-bound). Celebrate when you achieve them!

2. **Choose Activities You Enjoy**: You're more likely to stick with an exercise routine if you genuinely enjoy the activities. Whether it's hiking, cycling, yoga, or dancing, pick something that brings you joy.

3. **Establish a Routine**: Consistency is key. Try to set specific days and times for your workouts and make them as integral to your routine as eating or sleeping.

4. **Track Your Progress**: Keep a log of your activities and how you feel after doing them. Noting improvements in your mood and energy levels can be a significant motivator.

5. **Find an Exercise Buddy**: Working out with a friend can increase your motivation and make exercising more enjoyable. It's harder to skip a workout when someone is counting on you.

6. **Utilize Technology**: Fitness apps, online communities, or wearable technology can help keep you engaged and motivated. They can provide workout ideas, track your progress, and connect you with supportive communities.

7. **Reward Yourself**: After reaching a milestone, treat yourself to something enjoyable that doesn't contradict your goals (like a new book, a massage, or a special meal).

8. **Mix It Up**: Keep your routine interesting by trying different types of exercises. This not only prevents boredom but could also challenge different muscle groups and improve overall fitness.

9. **Focus on the Benefits**: Remind yourself how much better you feel after exercising, both physically and mentally. Keeping the benefits top of mind can motivate you to push through low-motivation periods.

10. **Listen to Your Body**: On days when you're feeling really down or tired, it's okay to take it easy. Sometimes, a gentle walk or some stretching is enough.

11. **Set up a Dedicated Space**: If possible, create a space that's dedicated to exercising. Having a set place can help to mentally prepare you for your workout.

12. **Join a Class or Group**: Being part of a class or an exercise group can offer social support and motivation.

Knowing others are expecting your participation can encourage attendance.

By implementing these strategies, you can maintain your motivation and enjoy the mental health benefits that regular exercise provides. Remember, the goal is to make exercise a part of your lifestyle—a component of your life that you miss when it's not there.

Certainly! Staying motivated in your fitness journey can be greatly supported by the right apps. Here are some versatile fitness apps that cater to various preferences and needs:

1. **MyFitnessPal**: Great for tracking diet and exercise, helping you maintain or achieve your fitness goals through calorie counting and nutrition insights.

2. **Strava**: Ideal for runners and cyclists, this app offers route planning, performance tracking, and a social aspect to share achievements with friends or join challenges.

3. **Fitbit**: Works best when paired with a Fitbit device, but it's also a solid standalone app for tracking activity, workouts, sleep, and nutrition.

4. **Nike Training Club**: Provides a wide range of workouts from strength training to yoga. It offers personalized training plans based on your goals and performance.

5. **Headspace**: While not a traditional fitness app, it's great for mental fitness, offering guided meditations, sleep sounds, and mindfulness exercises. A healthy mind is crucial for a healthy body.

6. **Peloton**: Known for its cycling classes, Peloton offers much more, including running, strength, yoga, and meditation classes. The app can be used with or without Peloton equipment.

7. **Zwift**: Combines video game elements with running and cycling workouts. It's highly engaging and allows you to interact with other users in a virtual world.

8. **JEFIT**: Perfect for strength training enthusiasts, JEFIT offers workout programs and the ability to track your training routines and progress.

9. **MapMyRun (by Under Armour)**: A comprehensive tool for runners, this app tracks and maps your runs, offers

personalized insights, and allows you to connect with a community.

10. **Daily Yoga**: Offers a vast library of yoga poses, guided classes, and meditation sessions suitable for all levels, from beginner to advanced.

Each of these apps has unique features that cater to different aspects of fitness, whether you're looking to track your nutrition, stay motivated with new workouts, connect with a community, or find peace of mind through meditation. Try a few to see which one aligns best with your goals and preferences.

Acknowledgements

First I would like to says all praises and thanks be to Allah, secondly I would like to thank my mother who birthed me and cultivated me and her loyalty late husband Donald C. Burrell who supported her and loved her and all 9 of the children they raised under one roof. I like to thank my Baby sister Spring for the most love and support over these past 14 years of my life because it's been tough at times but she stayed ten toes and always offered words of encouragement & her support! Next I would like to think brother Joe who's always had my back as well and never let me down but always help me stand tall while encouraging me to do better. I'ed also like to thank my oldest two brothers Rue & SQ who both has bestowed more blessings upon me than would ever be able to count, and they both have supported me & help me thru my struggles. I have to thank my three older sisters Nel, Del & Edy who have all been supportive and loving through out my entire existence & they all have inspired me & contributed to my growth and maturity in the most dynamical and beautiful ways! Of I would never leave out older brother Chill "the middle child" who was the one that showed me the most don'ts in life. I can't leave out my God parents and siblings who took me in from an infant til I was old enough to attend school. Aunt Liz & Uncle Charles words could never express my thanks enough! Shara & Worm y'all couldn't have loved me more…. So thank you all and the rest of the family and friends who supported me this far in life! The love and appreciation I have for my parents and family overflows like Niagara Falls! May Allaah guide us all & rectify our affairs. Allaahuma Ameen!

Short Autobiography of the author : Born James Daniel Green- Burrell June 3rd 1985 to Celeste and Donald Burrell in the beating heart of a bloody & unforgiving streets of Northeast Baltimore. With Seven other children my parents ended up allowing my mothers uncle and wife to help raise me as an alternative other than adoption. They raised me as their own and brought me up with the love care that a child nowadays could only hope for. When I was old enough to attend school it was agreed that I would be given back to my parents and I was, however by that time my parents had managed to have a whole nother baby! So I bounced back forth a while until finally I stayed with my parents full time. They raised me to be the best version of what they thought I could be…. But God had a plan too! After serving some time in prison I had begun to develop a habit of working out and reverted back to Islam. Now I have truly become the very best version of myself mentally physically and spiritually…. So I decided to share these gifts with the world especially those in need!

Sincerely,

James Burrell